Dr Sebi Approved Herbs

Using Dr Sebi Herbs to Naturally Cleanse and Cure the Body of All Diseases

Jack W. Roberts

Table of Contents

Disclaimer iii

Introduction 1

Anamu 3

Basil 6

Bay Leaf 11

Vervain 13

Burdock Root 15

Bugleweed 19

Blessed Thistle 24

Cascara Sagrada 28

Chickweed 33

Clove 36

Condurango 39

Contribo 42

Cordoncillo Negro 45

Dandelion 49

Dragon Tree 53

Elderberries 56

Eucalyptus 58

Fennel 62

Feverfew 67

Soursop 70

Conclusion 75

Disclaimer

Please note that the information in this book are written for the express purpose of sharing educational information only and it is stated to be reliable and consistence with the Dr Sebi healing style, but the author neither implies nor intends any guarantee of accuracy for specific cases or individuals as it is intended only as a general reference for further exploration.

It is recommended that you consult a licensed professional before beginning any practice relating to your health. The contents of this book are not replacement for professional health advice.

The author, publisher and distributors disclaim any liability, loss or damage and risk taken by individuals who directly or indirectly act on the information contained in this book.

Introduction

In several of his classes, Dr. Sebi emphasized the significance of using herbs to obtain the nutrients needed to combat any condition. He stated that it is impossible to become ill when the body receives the nutrients it requires to boost immunity and detox.

With the rise of various diseases presently, Dr. Sebi's recommendation is much more helpful than before. He was just as interested in preventing disease and illness as he was in treating them. Numerous people have seen Dr. Sebi's lectures and videos, in which he advised some essential herbal remedies that can greatly benefit our overall health. These botanicals are recognized for their capacity to dry up mucous, flush toxins from the body, and improve your immunity so you can fight disease effectively.

Although this isn't an exhaustive list, below are a few key herbs and regions of the body that Dr. Sebi advises to get you going.

Anamu

Parts Utilized: Entire herb

Anamu, called Petiveria alliacea in the science world, is a famous herbal plant with a variety of health benefits that assists the body to restore and deliver the required nutrients to combat various diseases and ailments. Although it originated from the Amazon forest and thrives in tropical climes, it may also be found in the Caribbean, Central America, and the southern United States.

Anamu's leaves, particularly its roots, have a pungent garlic-like smell, which is caused by active components in the shrub, mostly sulfur compounds. It is thought that the inclusion of numerous plant chemicals, such as lipids, triterpenes, flavonoids, sulfur, and coumarin compounds, is mostly liable for its health virtues. Also, Anamu is called guinea hen weed, guinea hen weed, guinea hen weed, guinea, apacin, and mucura.

Health Advantages

Traditional medicine practitioners have long utilized anamu to treat and manage a variety of chronic conditions, such as cancer. Although additional study is needed, animal and test-tube studies have connected anamu to the following health benefits:

- Due to the inclusion of triterpenes, flavonoids, sulfur compounds, coumarins, and other antioxidants, it might have antioxidant properties.

- It has the potential to relieve pain and inflammation.

- It has the potential to improve cognitive performance.

- It's possible that it has anti-cancer qualities. In colon, lung, breast, prostate, and pancreatic cancer cells, anamu preparations can help restrict cell growth and trigger apoptosis (programmed cell death).

- Could have antimicrobial activities.

- It has the potential to improve immunity.

- It has the potential to alleviate anxiety.

Basil

Parts Utilized: Essential oil, Leaf

Basils are tasty fragrant herbs that comes in a variety of types. It comes from Asia and Africa and is a member of the mint family. It's commonly utilized in cookery as a culinary flavoring, as well as in supplements and teas, and it could have a variety of health benefits.

Ocimum basilicum is the scientific name for the kind used in cookery. Also, it comes in a variety of flavors. They're as follows:

- **Sweet basil**: This is the most extensively produced and common basil, plus it is well-known for its usage in Italian cuisine. Dried versions are widely available at supermarkets. It tastes like licorice and cloves.

- **Greek or Bush basil**: These basil types have a very strong aroma and a moderate flavor and may be used in place of sweet basil. It grows nicely in a container and develops into a compact shrub with little leaves.

- **Thai basil**: This herb has a taste that is similar to anise-licorice and is often utilized in Southeast Asian and Thai cooking.

- **Cinnamon basil**: It originated from Mexico. It smells and tastes like cinnamon. Usually served with spicy, stir-fried veggies or legumes.

- **Lettuce basil**: This plant has huge, velvety, wrinkled leaves that have a taste similar to licorice. It's great in salads or mixed with tomatoes and olive oil.

Ocimum sanctum or Ocimum tenuiflorum is the scientific nomenclature for the basil frequently utilized in supplements and herbal-based tea. They're sometimes called tulsi or holy basil. Due to its particular flavor, it is used in various Thai recipes.

Health Advantages

Basil is indeed a common traditional therapy for nausea and insect bites, and it is also frequently utilized in Ayurvedic and traditional Chinese medical systems. Let's start by looking at the medical benefits of some of the commonest basil, which is used in supplements, tea, and cooking.

Sweet basil could be of assistance in:

- Preventing memory loss caused by stress and age.

- Relieving depression caused by long-term stress.

- Whether administered before or immediately after suffering a stroke, minimizes stroke harm and aids recovery.

- Augments triglycerides, cholesterol, and fasting blood sugar.

- Lower blood pressure in hypertensive patients. Aspirin-like effects thin the blood and dilate blood vessels.

- Prevent ulcers by protecting your gut from the effects of aspirin.

- Prevent malignancies of the pancreas, colon, and breast, among others.

- When breathed as aromatherapy, it boosts mental clarity.

- Prevents the germs that cause tooth decay from growing.

- Increase food safety, for example, if companies include it in food products.

- Provide a replacement for antibiotics in the treatment of contagious diseases, particularly in the fight against antibiotic-resistant bacterium strains.

- Repel insects, like ticks and mosquitos.

Holy Basil

While holy basil also has many of the same health benefits as its sweet basil counterpart, it's especially beneficial to diabetics. Its usefulness in decreasing blood sugar levels in type 2 diabetic patients has been demonstrated in research.

Bay Leaf

Parts Utilized: Leaf

Bay leaves are strong-flavored herbs that come from different plants and are commonly used in culinary preparations. Bay laurel trees are among the most well-known suppliers. Other bay leaf variations include:

- West Indian bay leaves
- Indonesian bay leaves
- California bay leaves
- Indian bay leaves
- Mexican bay leaves

These bay leave variants have a slightly distinct flavor. Bay leaves come in a variety of forms, including fresh, powdered, whole, and dried, rendering them a versatile culinary herb.

Health Advantages

- Bay leaves give flavor and improve the taste of foods without the addition of salts, which is good for the kidneys.
- Bay Leaves possess antioxidant and antimicrobial activities.
- Also, they've been utilized in the cure of dandruff, joint discomfort, and boils by certain individuals.
- Some people have utilized bay leaves for cancer treatment, but there isn't sufficient scientific data to support this.

Vervain

Parts Used: Leaf, Flower

Verbena Officinalis, sometimes called vervain, is a medicinal herb in the family of verbena herbs. Although there are more than two hundred and fifty different verbena species, vervain speaks of the ones utilized for medical purposes. Verbena hastata (blue vervain) and Verbena urticifolia (white vervain) are two less frequent varieties of Verbena Officinalis.

Health Advantages

Vervain can aid in the treatment of

- Headaches

- Insomnia and anxiety

- Relief from aches and pains in general

- Digestive problems

- Colorectal cancer

- Infections of the urinary tract

- Infectious illness that is both severe
  and common

- May aid in the prevention of kidney stones

- Symptoms of the upper respiratory tract

Burdock Root

Parts Utilized: Root

Burdock roots come from the burdock plant, a weed genus linked to sunflowers and a member of the family of daisy plants. It's known as gobo root in Japan and is grown as veggies. Burdock originated from North Asia and Europe, but it has become a weed in the U.S. Individuals in various regions of the globe eat it as root veggies, similar to potatoes and some other vegetables.

Burdock has big, purple-colored thistle-like to vivid pink-red flowers and heart-shaped leaves. Also, it possesses burrs that could cling to animal fur or clothes. On the exterior, the burdock's deep planted roots are greenish-brown to practically black.

Burdock roots are long, thin root veggies with brown skins that can grow to be more than two feet long. Volatile oils, carbohydrates, fatty oils, tannins, and plant sterols. Make up the majority of it.

Edible burdock, clotbur, bardana, great burdocks, Fructus arctii, Niu Bang Zi, lappa, big bur, and beggar's buttons are all names for burdock.

Health Advantages

Burdock root has a number of health benefits, including:

- Burdock roots are referred to as "blood purifiers" because they aid in the removal of toxins from the bloodstream and were thought to aid in the removal of toxins from the bloodstream.

- Burdock root aids in the detoxification of toxic metallic substances from the bloodstream, hence boosting organ and general wellbeing.

- Detoxification and lymphatic drainage are aided by burdock roots. They have a fantastic impact on the human lymphatic system due in part to their roles as natural blood cleaners. The human lymphatic system is the "drainage system" of the internal parts of the human body a web of lymph nodes and blood arteries that transport fluids from the body's tissues to the bloodstream and back. If you could strengthen your lymphatic system, it means that you can assist your system fight off a variety of ailments and major health problems.

- Its diuretic effects boost the kidneys, assisting in the removal of excessive amounts of fluid from your body, mostly water, and salt, and also waste products from your bloodstream.

- It enhances skin health by increasing blood flow towards the surface. Burdock root's topical products are supposed to treat a variety of skin disorders and improve skin health, plus aging symptoms.

- Protect against the onset of diabetes, particularly diabetic retinopathy, and aid digestion.

Bugleweed

Parts Utilized: Aerial parts

Bugleweed (also called Lycopus virginicus, scientifically) is a pungent-tasting, bitter fragrant plant with astringent qualities that are widely utilized in the treatment of thyroid issues. It is endemic to North America, with its origins in Europe. It may be found eastern part of the river Mississippi.

Bugleweed is an annual blooming species of the mint genus, although it does not have the minty scent that other mint variants have. Its rich purplish-blue blooms blossom to September from May (contingent on the region), and its seeds mature between July and September.

Bugleweed thrives in a variety of soil types (clay, loamy, and sandy) and pH ranges. It thrives in a damp climate and may grow rapidly in waterlogged soil. Its above-ground components (flowers and leaves) are used to make medicine.

Green archangel, Carpenter's herb, Bitter bugle, Paul's betony, Northern bugleweed, Gypsywort, Sweet bugle, Rough bugleweed, Purple archangel are all other names for bugleweed.

Health Advantages

- The occurrence of lithospermic acid, and other organic acids inside Bugleweed's extract such as lycopene, tannins, phenolic derivatives, and flavonoid glycosides, is thought to be responsible for bugleweed's therapeutic qualities.

- As a substitute for hormonal treatment, bugleweed is employed. Thyroxine and thyroid-stimulating hormone concentrations can be reduced by the plant's components. This impact might be related to the herbal drug's inhibitory effect on antibodies to the thyroid gland's binding.

- It's been utilized for centuries to prevent iodine transformation inside the thyroid gland. Hence, it can be utilized as a natural therapy for diseases such as hyperthyroidism.

- Bugleweed has historically been utilized to treat respiratory problems and coughs.

- It is utilized as one of the natural treatments methods for insomnia.

- In folk medicine, bugleweeds are utilized in the cure of cure heart palpitations, tuberculosis, and anxiety.

- Bugleweed extracts are supposed to help normalize heart rate, indicating that they might be used as an alternate therapy for tachycardia.

- The human sympathetic nervous system and vascular tissues are the principal targets of bugleweed extracts.

- Certain Grave's disease symptoms, like convulsions and palpitations, are treated naturally using bugleweed.

- Also, bugleweed leaves can be utilized to treat abrasions and wounds naturally.

Blessed Thistle

Parts Utilized: Aerial part

The blessed thistle, called Cnicus benedictus scientifically, is a hairy yearly plant that could reach a height of seventy centimeters. It has lanceolate leaves bearing a spiny border have a branchy stalk that is pentagonal in nature. The bright yellow blooms are grouped in a crest at the apex of the stalk. From May until August, the plant is in full flower.

It can be natively found in Southeast Asia and countries around the Mediterranean, but it may also be seen in Central Europe, the southern United States, and areas of Central and South America, both cultivated and wild. Due to their multiple medicinal properties, all of the herb's above-ground portions are employed in herbal therapy.

Also, blessed is called St. Benedict's thistle, Holy thistle, lady's thistle, sacred thistle blessed cardus, spotted cardo (Spanish), benediktenkraut cardin, (German), Chardon bénit (French).

Health Advantages

- Lignans, essential oils, tannins, and the minerals calcium, potassium, iron, magnesium, and manganese are all found in blessed thistle. Cnicin, the principal bitter component, is found in concentrations ranging from 0.2 - 0.7 percent.

- The plant was utilized in the treatment of malaria in Greek herbal medicine, and it was widely believed that it could also heal epidemic disorders including chickenpox, measles, plague, and smallpox.

- Indigestion, poor appetite, constipation, intestinal worms, respiratory disorders, colic, flatulence, anorexia, and diseases related to poor liver function such as irritability, weariness, and headache are all treated with the herb in herbal tea formulation.

- Blessed thistle's bitter ingredient (cnicin) stimulates hunger and improves digestion by increasing the release of digestive fluids from the stomach, salivary glands, bowels, gallbladder, and pancreas.

- The chemical cnicin, polyacetylene, and essential oil present in this plant have antibacterial effects.

- It might be utilized to boost immunity.

- It contains diuretic qualities, which might be beneficial in cases of high temperature or feverish situations.

- Being an expectorant, the plant can be utilized in the treatment of respiratory infections including flu and colds.

Cascara Sagrada

Parts Used: Bark

Cascara sagrada, called Rhamnus purshiana, scientifically, is a woody plant found in damp forests beneath five thousand feet in the American Northwest, stretching to the Alaska panhandle from northern California (1,500 m). Also, it is present in Montana and Idaho's Rockies. Before being used in laxative concoctions, the plant is gathered as quills and bark fragments and left to mature for a minimum of three hundred and sixty-five days.

Cascara sagrada must be matured for a minimum of one year before being utilized to decompose its anthrone compounds. The bark is a purgative if it isn't seasoned, and it'll produce severe vomiting and intestinal spasms. Heat can be used to age the plant artificially, however some valuable ingredients may well be destroyed. It has recently been utilized to flavor foods like candies, frozen dairy desserts, and baked goods, and is also a component of sunscreen products.

Right from the 1890s, this plant has been classified in the United States Pharmacopeia and has also been approved by the FDA (Food and Drug Administration) for utilization as over-the-counter laxatives. But, in November 2002, that clearance was revoked owing to concerns regarding cascara sagrada's long-term safeness and a paucity of efficacy studies.

Despite the FDA's offer to submit data, companies rejected owing to the expensive expense of clinical studies, opting instead to get their products redefined as "dietary supplements" instead of over-the-counter laxatives.

Cascara sagrada does not have to be mistaken for cascara, which is the dried peel of coffee cherries used in lattes and some other coffee beverages.

Alternative names for Cascara sagrada include Bearberry, California buckthorn, sacred bark, and yellow bark, as well as chitticum and chittem.

Health Advantages

- Cascara sagrada contains laxative properties and it could aid in the relief of constipation in certain individuals. Also, it is commonly utilized for problems with the digestive process.

- While some people believe that cascara sagrada can help treat or prevent gallstones, liver issues, hemorrhoids, fissures, and even cancer, there's not enough research data to back up these assertions.

- Cascara sagrada should only be used for a limited period of time. It is typically well-tolerated and safe when taken to treat periodic constipation. It may induce cramping and stomach discomfort in certain people (most commonly when utilized in the treatment

of serious constipation).

32

Chickweed

Parts Utilized: Entire herb

Chickweed, called Stellaria media, scientifically, is a yearly plant. It is a European native that's gotten indigenous in Northern America, where it is typically thought of as a weed. Chickweed is a strong and long-time traditional treatment regarded to provide substantial health advantages by alternative medicine professionals and herbalists.

Chickweed flowers, leaves, and stems have been utilized to prepare teas, extracts, and oral decoctions for eons. Chickweed is now more often utilized in the treatment of a number of skin diseases as a therapeutic ointment. While chickweed consumption is prevalent in certain cultures, it is usually avoided owing to the potential negative effects.

Chickweed is distinguished by its oval leaves, hairy stems, and daisy-like, small blooms with 5 crenelated petals; nevertheless, because of its toxicity, it is seldom consumed through the mouth. Notwithstanding its toxicity, the FDA (Food and Drug Administration) has not prohibited the use of chickweed, however, it is listed in the Food and Drug Administration Poisonous Plant Database.

Chicken wort, Maruns, Craches, Mouse ear, Starweed, Satin flower, Winterweed, and Tongue grass are some of the other names for it.

Health Benefits

- When used topically, chickweeds are thought to help with eczema, burns, psoriasis, rashes, itchy skin, and other skin disorders.

- Also, chickweeds can help with bowel issues, stomach problems, and constipation.

- Also, it can help with weight loss.

<u>Clove</u>

Parts Utilized: Undeveloped flower bud

Cloves, called Syzygium aromaticum, scientifically, are aromatic, dried flower buds with origins tracing to the Myrtaceae family evergreen tree endemic to Indonesia. Clove got its nomenclature from the Latin term "Clavus," meaning "nail."

Cloves are a common feature in gingerbread prepared products and important inclusion in lots of Indian cuisines. For the fragrance and aromatic flavor, these clove spikes that are "nail-like" have been driven into Oranges, Ham, and some other foods.

Cloves were utilized in some traditional medical preparations and they were also utilized as aromatic and sweet spices.

Health Advantages

- Cloves contain antibacterial characteristics, which means they can help halt the growth of germs and other microbes.

- Due to its capacity to control blood sugar, cloves could be beneficial in the treatment of diabetic patients.

- Cloves include chemicals that may aid to prevent ulcers in the stomach.

- Cloves include nutrients such as minerals, vitamins, and fiber, so adding crushed or whole cloves into your dish can supply certain critical nutrients.

- Cloves have been utilized to maintain a healthy respiratory and immune system because of their warming and digestion supporting qualities.

- Because of its impact on mouth bacteria, gingivitis, and plaque, clove oil might be utilized as a natural technique for keeping dental hygiene.

- Cloves are abundant in their composition of antioxidants, which help to protect cells from damage that can result in cancer.

Condurango

Parts Utilized: Bark, Vine

Condurango, called Marsdenia condurango, scientifically, is another South American asclepiadaceous vine that grows to be thirty feet and two feet wide. It is endemic to Ecuador. After sun drying its bark, it is hammered with the aid of a mallet to separate it from its stem.

It is sold as quilled sections that are two to four inches in length and half an inch in diameter. The surface is dark brown to pale greyish, almost smooth, roughened, and scaly, with several lenticels or warts, the scales are soft, longitudinally striate and inner side white brown; fracture granular, fibrous, short; odor mildly aromatic, particularly in fresh drug; taste aromatic and bitter.

Condurango Blanco, Common Condorvine, Eagle-Vine Bark, Condurango Cortex, Lechero, Gonolobus condurango, Marsdenia reichenbachii, Marsdenia condurango, Liane du Condor are some of the other names for this plant.

Health Advantages

- This plant has been touted as a cancer treatment that is effective in the initial stages but doesn't have any effect on the disease's progression.

- Condurango helps in the digestion process and also in the increase of appetite.

Contribo

Parts Utilized: Aerial part, Root

Aristolochia Grandiflora, called Aristolachia trilobites, scientifically, is a furry vine that thrives near streams and damp environments. It is endemic to Panama and southern Mexico. The leaves have a heart-shaped form and a tall stalk. Julia Morton characterized the blossom of the vine before it opened as matching the form of a duck, and the stalk resembling a beak and a thin tail drooping at the flip side, in her comprehensive compendium of flora life.

It has dark green leaves color with triple lobes, and the bark is tough and readily pulls off. Fresh plants' leaves burn in direct sunlight, showing that they have a low tolerance for it.

Every year from March to April, it blooms and bears seeds.

Contribo is frequently found in Traditional Chinese and Ayurvedic Medicine. Unlike several other herbs, this herb has a recorded medicinal history. has performed admirably

Duckflower, Trefle caraibe, hierba del Indio, Alcatraz, Calico Vine, Dutchman's Pipe, Pipe vegetale, Liana couresse, Tref, Twef, and Birthwort are some of the other names for this plant.

Health Advantages

- Contribo is utilized to boost energy, combat exhaustion, improve appetite and blood circulation, and boost immunity.

- Colds, flu, indigestion, constipation, stomach pains, depression, delayed periods, and type 2 diabetes are all treated with it.

- The leaves are used to treat snake and insect bites, as well as malaria, and they are used in the treatment of certain liver diseases.

- It works as an antidote to the venomous impacts of snake bites.

- It aids in the treatment of bladder stones, renal problems, and uterine problems, and is good for women who are pregnant.

Cordoncillo Negro

Parts Utilized: Bark

Piper aduncum, also called Cordoncillo negro, scientifically, is an alkaline and tropical plant that forms seeds that are efficiently dispersed by birds. These seeds sprout on their own and can take over native plants. Alkalinity is a lovely thing, however, hybridity is incapable of producing this wonderful event.

When a soldier of Spanish origin was injured in Peru, he found the virtues of the plant leaves and utilized them to halt the bleeding on his incisions. Europe, Central America, the Caribbean, and South America are all home to the plant.

Aperta-ruo, matico, cordoncillo, bamboo piper, erva-de-jaboti, erba di soldato, shiatani, santa Maria negro, spiky pepper, soldier's herb, soldaten cabbage are some of the other names for cordoncillo negro.

Health Advantages

- Cordoncillo negro is a herb that can be used to treat renal problems. It safeguards the liver and inhibits stones formation in the kidney.

- Cordoncillo negro can be utilized as a carminative and stomachic to help with digestion and removal of intestinal gas.

- It can be employed as an antiseptic for scrapes, cuts, wounds, boils, ulcers, mouthwash, and leech bites, among other things.

- Also, it can be utilized in the treatment of stomach discomfort, nausea, vomiting, dysentery, dyspepsia, and dyspepsia.

- Cordoncillo negro is a hemostat that can be utilized to stop internal bleeding (pulmonary, gastric, uterine)

- Cordoncillo negro, as an antibiotic, can be utilized to treat infections caused by bacteria.

- Cordoncillo negro can be used to treat sexual dysfunction and genitourinary tract infections.

- Syphilis, gonorrhea, and some other STDs can all be treated with Cordoncillo negro

- Cordoncillo negro is a plant that can be used for the treatment of flu, colds, pneumonia, bronchitis, coughs, and other respiratory issues.

Dandelion

Parts Utilized: Leaf, Root

Dandelion called Taraxacum species, scientifically, is a floral plant that grows in various regions of the globe. It's an annual plant that may reach a height of eighteen inches. It thrives in rosettes near the ground and has dark greenish leaves with serrated margins. It features yellow blooms that open once it is morning and close towards the onset of evening, staying shut all through the night and on rainy days. Dandelion is a simple to grow plant that loves wet soil and direct sunlight.

The dandelion herb is said to have arisen from Central Asia, from whence it spread to semi-tropical and temperate regions across the world, plus the Mediterranean. It's a resilient plant that may be found growing wild in meadows, lawns, and fields.

While most people would consider dandelion (Taraxacum officinale) to be a tenacious weed, it's long been utilized in herbal formulations to assist digestion and promote appetite. The whole dandelion plant, from blossom to root, is edible and has a somewhat bitter, chicory-like flavor.

Cankerwort, Blowball, Priest's Crown, Lion's Tooth, Wild Endive, Swine Snout, Piss in-Bed, Fairy Clock, and Canker Wart are all names for the same plant.

Health Advantages

- Because of the occurrence of several bioactive substances such as polyphenols inside the plant, dandelion could be useful in lowering inflammation induced by illness.

- Dandelion's bioactive components may reduce cholesterol, lowering the risk of cardiovascular disease.

- Some individuals believe that dandelion can help lower blood pressure, although there isn't much data to back this up.

- May aid in the maintenance of a robust liver as well as immune function.

- Dandelion can be utilized in the treatment of constipation and some other digestive problems.

- Dandelion contains two beneficial compounds: chlorogenic and chicoric acid.

They might be present in all sections of the herb and might aid with blood sugar control.

- Inulin, a carbohydrate, which is present in plants and stimulates the establishment and upkeep of a robust bacterial population in our digestive system, is abundant in the dandelion's roots.

Dragon Tree

Parts Utilized: Bark, Leaf

The dragon tree, also called Dracaena marginata, scientifically, is a beautiful, stiff-leaved shrub endemic to Mauritius and Madagascar with sword-like greenish leaves bordered with crimson. The plant features short, gray slender stems that are crowned with sword-shaped, gleaming leaves. The fragrant little white flowers emerge in the springtime on the exterior variety, accompanied by round orange-yellow berries. Plant resins have been utilized for a variety of applications for quite some time. It was used by the ancient Romans and Greeks, as well as in the Middle East, India, and China.

In warm exterior settings, this little tree may reach a height of twenty feet, however, it is most commonly cultivated as a planted houseplant with a height of six feet or even less. It can withstand a broad variety of temperatures, unlike what's obtainable with several indoor trees. Drought-proof plants with vigorous root systems, dragon trees make great houseplants. It is sometimes cultivated as a sole-stemmed plant, and sometimes they're clustered or knotted in groups inside a pot.

Also, this tree is called the Draco dragon plant, Dracaena, and Drago.

Health Advantages

- Dragon plants contain antibacterial qualities and may provide some safety from infections such as viruses, fungus, and bacteria, or even destroy them.

- The dragon herb has been utilized for healthy digestion since ancient times. The plant resins were utilized to cure dysentery and diarrhea in particular.

- Dragon's blood might assist with topical ulcers, however, the evidence isn't yet conclusive. Its antibacterial qualities may account for its topical benefit. However, it is not a substitute for doctor-advised therapeutic methods.

Elderberries

Parts Utilized: Flowers, Berries

The elderberry shrub purple-colored fruit is known as elderberries (Sambucus spp). The most prevalent kind is Sambucus nigra, which is high in antioxidants called anthocyanins. Miniature whitish or creamy elderflower bunches and clusters of small black or blue elderberries adorn the tree. Elderberries have long been employed by European herbalists and Native Americans for their alleged health advantages.

Baises de Sureau, Ellenwood, Black Elderberry, Black Elder, Boor Tree, Baccae, Elder, Bountry, Black-Berried Alder, and Common Elder are all names for elderberries.

Health Advantages

- Elderberry is utilized in the treatment of the common cold, influenza (the flu), and swine flu. it is utilized to help the body's immunological system.

- Elderberry can help with nasal discomfort, nerve pain, leg and back pain, and CFS (chronic fatigue syndrome).

- Elderberry is used to treat constipation, cancer, hay fever, boost urine output, and produce sweating in certain individuals.

- Elderberry is used to treat gum irritation within the mouth.

- It's utilized to treat high cholesterol, heart disease, weight reduction, toothaches, and headaches, among other things.

Eucalyptus

Parts Utilized: Leaf

Eucalyptus, called Eucalyptus globulus, scientifically, this plant is a grown evergreen plant endemic to Australia. In the parched desert, it was initially employed by the Aborigines, who consumed the roots because they contain a high concentration of water. They used eucalyptus tea for fever cure. Eucalyptus gained popularity as one of the foremost Australian fever tea as its use grew.

Dating back to 1788, when physicians noticed the existence of the oil and started utilizing it to cure colic and chest ailments, the supersaturated oil steam extracted from the tree's leaves has been utilized medicinally. Eucalyptus oil was given for respiratory problems such as flu, bronchitis, coughs, and asthma towards the end of the late 1800s owing to its capacity to increase perspiration and remove mucus.

As news of eucalyptus oil grew, it was utilized for a variety of purposes, often as liniments for fatigued, painful muscles and also to relieve arthritic pain. Although this essential oil was used for a variety of therapeutic purposes, it is most commonly used to treat bronchitis, colds, coughs, and symptomatic relief from colds and upper respiratory congestion.

Health Advantages

- Eucalyptus leaves are high in antioxidants, especially flavonoids, which safeguard the body from damages caused by free radicals and oxidative stress, perhaps lowering your risk of dementia, heart disease, and cancer.

- Eucalyptus oil has been linked to lower anxiety and blood pressure. The parasympathetic nervous system (PNS), which facilitates relaxation, is thought to be activated by it.

- The component eucalyptol found in eucalyptus oil has been proved to put off mosquitoes and some other insects that bite. It might potentially be a helpful head lice treatment, but additional study is required.

- Chewing gum that has leaf extracts from eucalyptus has been shown to reduce plaque accumulation on teeth and gum disease symptoms.

- Extract from Eucalyptus has been demonstrated to treat dandruff and dry skin by increasing ceramide formation in the skin. This needs to be confirmed by more studies.

Fennel

Parts Utilized: Seed

Fennels are fragrant, perennial plants with yellow blooms. It's originally from the Mediterranean, however, it is now found all across the globe. The bulb is pale, and the stalks are tall and greenish. It can thrive in practically any environment. The stalk, bulb, seeds, and leaves are all edible portions of the plant.

The fennel bulb is a source of energy, potassium, dietary fiber, vitamin C, and other critical minerals including salt, phosphorus, and calcium, as per the USDA National Nutrient Database for Standard Reference. Iron, magnesium, zinc, niacin, and vitamin K are all present at modest levels. Beta carotene,

B vitamins, vitamin A, and flavonols are also present.

Being a spice flavored with anise, dried fennel seeds are commonly used in cookery. But do not mix fennel and anise; they aren't identical, even if they taste and look alike. The oil and dried mature seeds of the fennel plant are employed in the formulation of the medication.

Also, Fennel is known by the names Almindelig Fennikel, Adas, Anethum piperitum, Anethum Foeniculum, Badishep, Badian, Arapsaci, Bitterfenchel, Bisbas, Bari Sanuf, Common Fennel, Carosella, Bitter Fennel, Erva-doce, Endro, Dunkler Fenchel, Fennel Seed, Fenchle, Fenchel, F

Health Advantages

- Because some constituents of fennel, including cineole and anethol, have disinfecting and antibiotic qualities, they can help treat diarrhea due to bacterial infections.

- Fennel is high in numerous nutrients, notably vitamin C, which helps to strengthen immunity and protects the body from damage from free radicals and infection.

- Because of the carminative qualities of the amino acid present in fennel, it is often used in an anti-flatulence procedure. Several people, from newborns to geriatrics, can benefit from its extract to decrease flatulence and remove excessive gas from the gut.

- Fennel seeds, especially when powdered, are regarded to have laxative properties in Ayurvedic medicine. Roughage aids in colon cleansing, while its stimulating impact aids in maintaining correct peristaltic activity inside the intestines, which aids in excretion.

- Fennel aids in the maintenance of good cholesterol concentrations inside the bloodstream. What this means is that it can help the body get rid of harmful bad cholesterol that has been linked to strokes, atherosclerosis, and heart disease.

- Both the amino acid histidine and iron contained inside the fennel plant, are beneficial in the treatment of anemia. The amino acid histidine and iron positioned at number fifteen of the hemoglobin complex drives hemoglobin development, the primary histidine aids in the development of numerous other blood components.

- Also, Fennel is an emmenagogue, meaning that it is supposed to help regulate and relieve menstruation by balancing the hormones responsible for that. Regulating the body's hormonal activity.

Feverfew

Parts Utilized: The whole plant

Feverfew, called Tanacetum parthenium, scientifically, is a sunflower family flowering plant (Asteraceae family). The term febrifugia stems from the Latin term febrifugia, which means "fever reducer." This is a plant that originated in the Balkans and Asia Minor but is currently found all across the globe.

In European traditional medicine, feverfew has traditionally been utilized as natural medicine. Its leaves are typically dried for usage, although extracts and fresh leaves are indeed available. It includes parthenolide, a chemical that may aid to decrease inflammation, relieve muscular spasms, and prevent blood vessel constriction inside the brain. This plant is alternatively called Altamisa, Wild Chamomile, Featherfew, Chrysanthemum parthenium, Chrysanthème Matricaire, Bachelor's Buttons, Featherfoil, Featerfoiul, Chrysanthemum praealtum, Leucanthemum parthenium, Grande Camomille, Flirtwort Midsummer Daisy, Chrysanthemum praealtum, Leucanthem

Health Advantages

- Studies suggest that eating feverfew decreases the incidence of migraines and helps to eliminate symptoms such as nausea, discomfort, headaches, vomiting, and intolerance to noise and light.

- Feverfew extract creams without parthenolide may assist in combating acne rosacea by lowering inflammation. Because parthenolide might cause skin irritation, it's not used in topical treatments.

- Feverfew was shown to help lessen sadness and anxiety symptoms in animal experiments. Human research in this area, however, is not known.

- Feverfew chemicals possess anti-cancer effects and might suppress specific cancer cells, according to several test-tube research.

Soursop

Parts Utilized: Leaf

Soursop, also called Annona muricata, is among the custard apple tree family (Annonaceae) that is planted for its enormous eatable fruits. The tree is endemic to the American tropics, but it has spread far across the tropical regions of the Old World. The evergreen leaves of the soursop tree are broad-ended ovals that are about five inches in length. The fragrant fruits are oval-shaped, spiky, as well as green-skinned, with a length of around eight inches and a weight of up to 4.5 kilograms. The species is often grown as a seed and thrives in warmer environments with towering humidity.

The fibrous whitish flesh of the fruit, which has pineapple and mango flavors, may be eaten raw or strained to produce cocktails, ice creams, and custards.

Guanabana, Brazilian pawpaw, and Graviola are all other names for soursop.

Health Advantages

- The anti-inflammatory qualities of soursop can assist individuals with respiratory disorders including colds, coughs, and other kinds of congestion unclog their passageways, reduce inflammation, and alleviate congestion. Consuming soursop is an effective technique to get rid of mucus and phlegm, which can harbor a variety of diseases.

- Including a little amount of soursop fruit inside your diet, whether in sweets or delightful beverages, can benefit your general health. The soursop's high vitamin C content encourages the development of white blood cells, whereas its high antioxidant content helps stop the onset of chronic illness and scavenge free radicals.

- Because of its anti-inflammatory and analgesic effects, soursop is well-known as a painkiller. It's been used to treat injuries and wounds for centuries and has been shown to be effective.

- On the inside, to hasten healing and alleviate discomfort. This fruit's anti-inflammatory properties render it an excellent treatment for a variety of ailments.

- If you are having trouble sleeping or have insomnia, this plant is a good option. It's been utilized as a way to unwind for ages. Soursop has calming and anti-inflammatory qualities that render it particularly useful for people who suffer from anxiety and stress.

- The organic constituents of soursop have been extensively researched, and it's been intensively examined as an alternate cancer therapy. Its antioxidant property, which is derived from acetogenins, and also alkaloids, and quinolones, has been associated with preventing cancer and tumor shrinkage. They've been linked to the treatment of pancreatic, breast, lung, and prostate cancers due to their ability to

shut off blood circulation to alien or non-

regular cellular developments.

Conclusion

These herb lists are in line with Dr. Sebi's approach of employing herbs for a variety of ailments due to their medicinal benefits. Dr. Sebi either mentions them or includes them in many of his products.

However, it is not recommended that these plants be consumed by children.

- Children under the age of twelve should not take it.
- Expectant mothers (pregnant women) should avoid it as well.

That's owing to a dearth of evidence on the effects of most botanicals on pregnant women, children, and infants. Certain herbs have even been proven to be harmful to expectant mothers, therefore it is better for them to avoid them entirely.

It's also worth noting that, although these herbs offer a variety of health advantages, many of them still require additional scientific research to support certain of their applications for specific ailments. As a result, using these medicines under the guidance of a certified healthcare professional, such as a naturopathic specialist, is recommended.